MARKED BY HISTORY

by Cathy R. Foreman

MaeCarol
PRESS

Published by MaeCarol Press

First Edition

ISBN 979-8-9930292-2-1

Good and evil are not assigned by skin.

They exist in all people.

The true enemy has always been ignorance…

And still is.

~ Cathy

A Note on Perspective

Ignorance is not the absence of knowledge.
It is the refusal to see.

It lingers in the spaces between memory and action... in the choices we inherit, and in the blind spots we learn to live with.
It shows up in what is remembered, what is erased, and what is quietly passed down as truth.

This book is my attempt to trace those lines.
To look honestly at the ways identity, heritage, and medicine collide.
And to ask the questions we tend to avoid - the ones that unsettle what we think we know.

This is not a neutral book.
Not by any means.

It does not hide, soften, or apologize.

But it is curious.
Honest.
Stubborn.

It moves slowly where it needs to
and presses where it must.

It is both a mirror and a map:
a reflection of how we've been marked...

and a guide through how we survive and reclaim what was denied.

What follows is not a comprehensive history or an academic record.
It is a gathering of threads - stories, research, observations, and lived experience - woven together to reveal patterns often ignored or dismissed.

Some of these patterns are familiar.
Others may feel uncomfortable - even confrontational.

That discomfort is not incidental.
It is part of the work.

This has been building over time.

Stories that stayed with me.
Encounters that felt incidental at first... but weren't.
Questions - some rooted in my own experience, others handed to me without warning - that refused to settle.

The more I followed the threads - across communities, across time, across bodies - the more I learned.
And the harder it became to ignore how often these stories are minimized, fragmented, or explained away.

Writing this book became less about having answers and more about refusing silence where curiosity was required.

You will encounter stories that unsettle...
details that linger...
truths that refuse comfort.

Pause.
Question.
Lean in.

Sit with what resists easy answers.
Sit with what challenges the narratives we've been taught to accept without interrogation.

I don't offer conclusions neatly tied in a bow.
I offer a lens: a way to pause, to question, to see more clearly.

The hope is that by stepping into this perspective, you'll find your own connections:
to your past...
to the legacies that shape us...
and to the courage it takes to name them and carry them differently.

Read with care.
Read with curiosity.

And read with the audacity to face what history asks you to confront.

~Cathy

What Remains

This book is not an argument against medicine.
Nor is it an attempt to relitigate history.

It is an exploration of what history leaves behind:
in systems, in families, in perception, in trust... and in the body itself.

Because sometimes what looks like fear, hesitation, silence, or resistance is not born in the present moment at all.

Sometimes it is inherited.

Sometimes the body remembers what the records forgot.

And for many people, especially Black Americans, the records were incomplete to begin with.

Names changed. Histories were interrupted. Origins blurred. Stories were withheld for survival. Entire lineages were broken by displacement, violence, silence, and time.

We are often asked to understand our bodies through systems that expect clarity... while carrying histories shaped by absence.

Family medical histories go missing. Cultural context disappears. Baselines are generalized. Identity is reduced to categories broad enough to fit a form but too narrow to explain a life.

This book lives in those gaps, asking what happens when inherited memory, historical harm, fractured lineage, and modern systems collide - quietly shaping trust, behavior, care, perception, and the ways people move through the world.

Not everything carried is visible.
Not everything inherited is spoken.

But absence leaves marks too.

CONTENTS

Introduction - The Form in Front of Me

Going to the doctor shouldn't feel like taking a statistics test, especially as a new patient. A form in front of me, and suddenly I'm expected to know everything about my body... and everybody else's, too.

Now that I'm older, there's always some damn form to fill out - new doctor, new health concern, insurance changes. Sometimes it's for me, sometimes it's for my mom. Then they want family medical history: heart disease, kidney disease, ocular issues... from both sides of the family. And if you can, they want dates. Dates! Like I sat around my grandma's kitchen table memorizing the exact year my great-grandfather had high blood pressure. Spoiler alert: I didn't even know my great-grandfather.

Add in a Black American family context where relationships can be fractured or nonexistent, along with parents who didn't talk about their own parents... and boom. You're staring at blank spaces and wondering: what the hell do I even put here?

Does not knowing this stuff matter for my health? For my risk? For my future? The truth is... it does. Black Americans are statistically more likely to develop hypertension, diabetes, and kidney disease, yet for many of us, the very history that might help prevent or catch these conditions early is hidden, incomplete, or simply unasked.

This book isn't only about the medical histories we inherit, but the ones we're denied - and the ones we must also reclaim.

Then there's my mom. I go to her appointments so I can "stay in the know," making sure she's telling the doctors everything. When I ask her questions, she shrugs. "I. Don't. Know." Classic, attitudinal Mary. So, we muddle through with what little information we have, piecing together fragments like some DIY ancestry puzzle.

The form in front of me wasn't new. It was simply the latest version of record-keeping that had always been incomplete.

And it hits me: this isn't just about forms. It's about a history of gaps. Gaps left by families who didn't talk about illness. By systems that didn't track us properly. By a culture that taught us to survive without asking too many questions.

That's how this book started. A personal journey that kept unfolding, stretching beyond me into a larger truth. A pull-back-the-covers moment that forced me to explore Black American history, our complicated relationship with doctors, and the quiet silences that live in our families, the grown folks' business we were never meant to know.

To understand my health, I had to understand my history. Not the one written in textbooks, but the one written in my blood.

And that's the part no one prepares you for.
That understanding your body might mean confronting things no one ever explained... or maybe never knew how to.

Because sometimes what we inherit isn't just risk.

It's silence.

The Missing Link

Not everything we inherit has a name.

Some things show up first.

Explanation comes later.

The missing chart isn't just a form. It exists in our bodies, blood, memory, and identity. Identity isn't just who we say we are;
it's what we've been shaped by, what we've inherited, and what we were never told.

Every medical form reminds me: it's not enough to know my own body. I have to know the history I wasn't given. I have to ask questions I was taught not to ask.

I remember the phrase clearly: "That's grown folks' business."
Back then, maybe it was. Now? Now it's mine. What I didn't realize then was that the silence wasn't just cultural. It was structural.
And those are not the same.

Doctors aren't asking out of curiosity. They're trying to predict what may already be moving through my bloodline before it shows up in my body. But prediction requires information. And for many of us, that information was never passed down, never recorded, or never explained.

And here's the part nobody really talks about:

Identity.

Not identity as a checkbox.

Identity as inheritance.

What's in your bloodline that never made it into conversation?

What doesn't show up on paperwork, but absolutely shows up in risk?

Not everything that matters *gets* written down.

And not everything that's written down...

tells the truth.

Every family carries stories that were softened, shortened, or swallowed. Those omissions shape our health as much as our DNA.

That's the missing link: the space between what was lived, what was recorded, and what was never explained.

Understanding cultural identity isn't just about pride.
It's about survival. It's about truth.
It's about putting all the pieces on the table, even the ones we were taught not to ask about.

The record exists.
The story doesn't always follow.

The Gaps We Inherit

The record tells a story.

Just not the whole story.

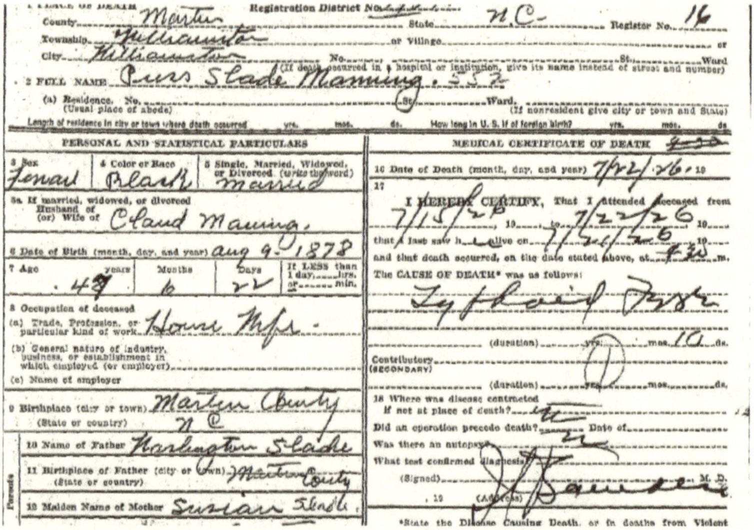

PLACE OF DEATH
County Martin Registration District No. State N.C. Register No. 16
Township Williamston or Village or
City Williamston No. St. Ward (If death occurred in a hospital or institution, give its name instead of street and number)
2 FULL NAME Puss Slade Manning. 552
(a) Residence. No. St. Ward. (Usual place of abode) (If nonresident give city or town and State)
Length of residence in city or town where death occurred yrs. mos. ds. How long in U. S. if of foreign birth? yrs. mos. ds.

PERSONAL AND STATISTICAL PARTICULARS
3 Sex Female 4 Color or Race Black 5 Single, Married, Widowed, or Divorced (write the word) married
5a If married, widowed, or divorced Husband of (or) Wife of Claud Manning.
6 Date of Birth (month, day, and year) aug 9 - 1878
7 Age years 47 Months 6 Days 22 If LESS than 1 day, hrs. or min.
8 Occupation of deceased (a) Trade, Profession, or particular kind of work House Wife.
(b) General nature of industry, business, or establishment in which employed (or employer)
(c) Name of employer
9 Birthplace (city or town) Martin County (State or country) N C
10 Name of Father Harlington Slade
11 Birthplace of Father (city or town) (State or country) Martin County
12 Maiden Name of Mother Susian Slade

MEDICAL CERTIFICATE OF DEATH
16 Date of Death (month, day, and year) 7/22/26
17 I HEREBY CERTIFY, That I attended deceased from 7/15/26, 19 to 7/22/26, 19
that I last saw h alive on 7/22/26 19
and that death occurred, on the date stated above, at 4 30 m.
The CAUSE OF DEATH* was as follows:
Typhoid Fever
(duration) yrs. mos. 10 ds.
Contributory (SECONDARY)
(duration) yrs. mos. ds.
18 Where was disease contracted if not at place of death?
Did an operation precede death? Date of
Was there an autopsy?
What test confirmed diagnosis?
(Signed) M. D.
, 19 (Address)
*State the Disease Causing Death, or in deaths from Violent

Death Certificate of my great-great grandmother, Puss Slade Manning, listing Typhoid Fever as her cause of death

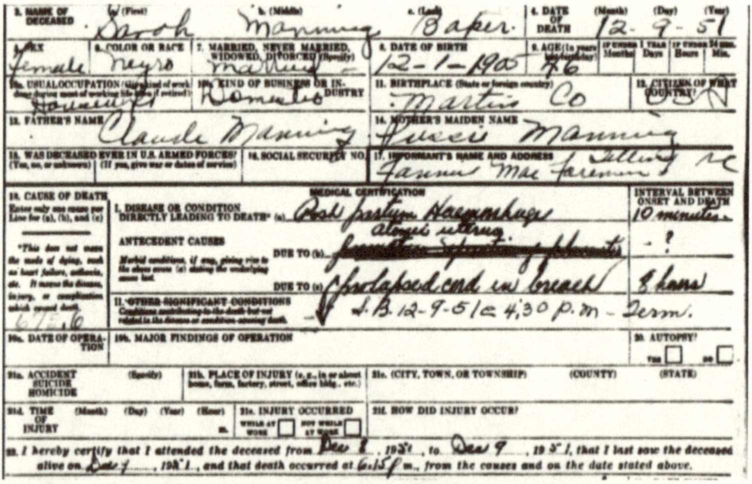

1. NAME OF DECEASED	a. (First) Sarah	b. (Middle) Manning	c. (Last) Baker	4. DATE OF DEATH	(Month) 12	(Day) 9	(Year) 51
5. SEX Female	6. COLOR OR RACE negro	7. MARRIED, NEVER MARRIED, WIDOWED, DIVORCED (Specify) married	8. DATE OF BIRTH 12-1-1905	9. AGE (In years last birthday) 46			
10a. USUAL OCCUPATION Housewife	10b. KIND OF BUSINESS OR INDUSTRY Domestic	11. BIRTHPLACE (State or foreign country) Martin Co	12. CITIZEN OF WHAT COUNTRY? USA				
13. FATHER'S NAME Claude Manning	14. MOTHER'S MAIDEN NAME Pussie Manning						
15. WAS DECEASED EVER IN U.S. ARMED FORCES?	16. SOCIAL SECURITY NO.	17. INFORMANT'S NAME AND ADDRESS Fannie Mae Foreman					

18. CAUSE OF DEATH — MEDICAL CERTIFICATION
I. DISEASE OR CONDITION DIRECTLY LEADING TO DEATH* (a) Post partum Haemmhage atonic uterus — INTERVAL BETWEEN ONSET AND DEATH: 10 minutes
ANTECEDENT CAUSES — DUE TO (b) ~~[illegible]~~ — ?
DUE TO (c) prolapsed cord in breach — 8 hours
II. OTHER SIGNIFICANT CONDITIONS — S.B. 12-9-51 @ 4:30 p.m. - Term.
19a. DATE OF OPERATION 19b. MAJOR FINDINGS OF OPERATION 20. AUTOPSY? YES ☐ NO ☐
21a. ACCIDENT SUICIDE HOMICIDE (Specify) 21b. PLACE OF INJURY 21c. (CITY, TOWN, OR TOWNSHIP) (COUNTY) (STATE)
21d. TIME OF INJURY (Month) (Day) (Year) (Hour) m. 21e. INJURY OCCURRED WHILE AT WORK ☐ NOT WHILE AT WORK ☐ 21f. HOW DID INJURY OCCUR?
22. I hereby certify that I attended the deceased from Dec 8, 1951, to Dec 9, 1951, that I last saw the deceased alive on Dec 9, 1951, and that death occurred at 6:15 p m., from the causes and on the date stated above.

Death Certificate of my great-grandmother, Sarah Manning Baker, listing Post Partum Hemorrhage as her cause of death

Before we talk about health, we have to talk about what was never explained.

Because the record is often the only thing that survives... and even then, it rarely tells the whole truth.

Puss Slade Manning died in 1926.
Cause of death: Typhoid.
The informant: her husband.

Twenty-five years later...

Sarah Manning Baker died in 1951.
Cause of death: Postpartum hemorrhage. Due to uterine complications. Due to a breech birth.
The informant: her eldest daughter... my grandmother, just twenty-three years old.

Mother and daughter.

I didn't begin with their stories. I began with their paperwork.

It wasn't just what was written that got to me...

it was how much was missing.

Two certificates. Two generations. Two deaths reduced to a handful of lines: names, dates, causes.

Enough to file. Enough to close a record.

Not enough to understand a life… or its ending.

Puss's death is attributed to typhoid.

A word that sounds precise. Clinical. Final.

But the document offers no explanation: no source, no conditions, no context. Just the diagnosis, written as if naming it were the same as understanding it.

Precision without context is its own kind of erasure.

Sarah's certificate tries harder.

Postpartum hemorrhage. Uterine complications. A breech birth. An interval measured in minutes.

As a whole, it attempts to sound explanatory. More ink. More effort.

And still… no account of care. No indication of urgency, delay, or response.

The outcome is documented.

The decisions are not.

Between these two women, mother and daughter, medicine advanced. Forms expanded. Language improved.

What remained unchanged was who was left to account for what happened.

The records were complete enough to file. Yet the gaps remained.

While the certificates clearly denote who reported the deaths, they do not ask who explained what happened, or when. They do not ask whether the informants witnessed the events, inferred details afterward, or simply repeated what they were told. They do not ask how medical language was understood or absorbed by those left behind.

They do, however, ask for certainty...

or at least the appearance of it.

Typhoid fever.

Postpartum hemorrhage.

The terms are firm.

The context is not.

In both cases, the informants were immediate family members. Close enough to validate the record. Not necessarily included in the decisions that preceded the outcome.

Reading these documents decades later, it was clear there was room for more detail.

But... it went unused.

Whether the information was unknown to the informants or simply unimportant to the record, once a cause was named...

the record closed.

Silence, it seems, was a sufficient ending.

For my grandmother, that silence arrived early.

At twenty-three, she was expected to confirm her mother's death using language she did not author and likely did not fully understand.

The form required a kind of accuracy.

Not comprehension.

And when comprehension is missing, the story that gets passed down is already incomplete.

As the story moved forward through the family, details softened. Simplified. Or were never spoken at all.

Not because they were intentionally withheld,

but because no one had ever been asked to explain them.

The form did not uncover forgotten information. It revealed information that had never been fully transmitted because, so little had ever been explained.

What remained was the official version:

brief, authoritative, and incomplete.

Decades later, in a doctor's office, I was handed a clipboard.

The questions felt familiar.

Family history. Medical background. Ancestry.

Checkboxes and short lines, designed for efficiency.

The form did not ask how certain the answers were. It did not ask how the information had been passed down...

or what had been omitted along the way.

It assumed continuity.

But continuity requires transmission.

And transmission requires explanation.

What these forms do not account for is how often medical information enters a family through stories, or only at its endpoint: through death certificates, discharge summaries, or final diagnoses, without ever being explained in a way that can be carried forward intact.

Over time, that matters.

Details become approximations.

Medical terms become shorthand.

Context thins.

Not because families are careless...

but because they are asked to preserve information that was never fully shared with them to begin with.

This is not a failure of memory.

It is a failure of transmission.

Information was passed. Just not fully. Just not clearly.

Just enough to close the record.

Not enough to carry the truth.

The gaps were not dramatic.

They were procedural.

They occurred at moments designed for closure... not conversation.

But procedural gaps become generational gaps when no one explains what happened.

The record needed to be finished.

The form needed to be completed.

Explanation... not required.

So, when someone hesitates over a family history question, or answers "unknown," it is not always uncertainty.

Sometimes it is accuracy.

Sometimes it is an honest reflection of what was never spoken or clarified. Only recorded.

And these small silences sit on top of much older ones…

the ones created by systems, not families.

The gaps did not begin with me.

But I am the one now standing in front of the form.

Before there was proof,

there was knowing.

And knowing kept people alive.

Night Doctors

In the dark, they took us....

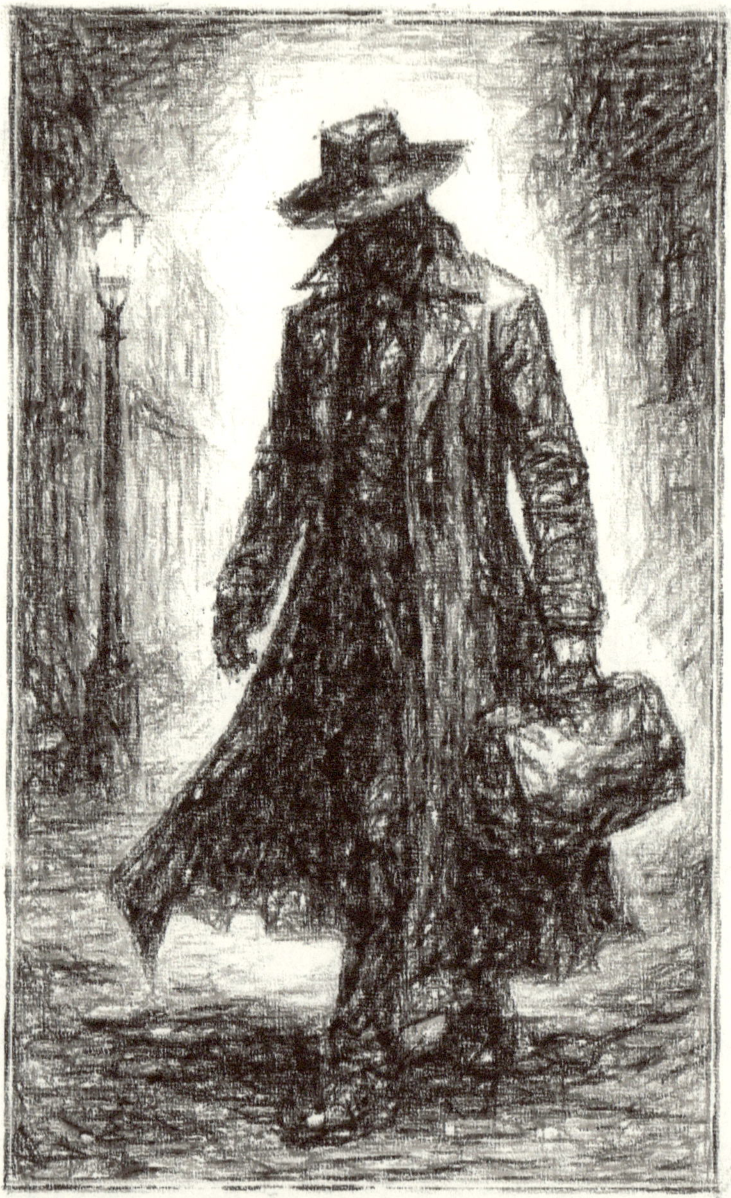

Illustration of a "Night Doctor"

The Sound That Stopped Me

I was in another room, half-listening, channel surfing, trying to figure out what I was going to watch next. You know that distracted way you do when the TV is running in more than one room and none of it really has your attention. My mom had a show on when a single line cut through the noise and made me stop.

I muted my TV.

What I heard... *night doctors.*

I didn't know the term, but my reaction to it was equal parts curiosity and alarm. I listened closer, and a moment later I walked into the other room and copped a squat.

As I settled in, I realized she was watching Law & Order, the original. The episode felt familiar, like I'd seen this story before... or at least pieces of it.

It felt like a take on Henrietta Lacks' story.

The episode was more than halfway through, so I pulled up the guide, planning to circle back later and watch it from the beginning. The title stopped me.

"Immortal."

Some words don't just describe. They reveal. And this one felt intentional... A synchronicity that, aside from validating my read of the storyline, felt like further confirmation that I was exactly where I was supposed to be with this project.

They were talking about *night doctors*. About blood. About cells taken from a family and used for decades, without their knowledge or meaningful permission, for research, treatments, cures, and breakthroughs.

The kind of scientific progress we celebrate without asking too many questions about where it came from.

It was familiar.

I grabbed my phone and looked it up. Sure enough - ripped from the headlines. A fictionalized retelling of the Henrietta Lacks story. Her cells. HeLa. Taken without consent. Replicated endlessly. Profitable. Lifesaving. Completely detached from the woman they came from.

I already knew this story. Most of us do now.

But this time, a shadow of a detail lingered.

Night doctors... a term unfamiliar to me.

It wasn't said dramatically - no ominous music cue. Just a reference slipped into the dialogue as if it were common knowledge. As if no explanation was needed.

And that's what caught me.
How quickly the story grew beyond Henrietta - bigger than one woman, one hospital, one mistake.

In the context of the journey I was already on, it opened into something older… broader.
A story with deeper roots and heavier implications.

A more deliberate history.

The question shifted.

Not *what happened to her?*

But *how long had this been happening, and who already knew?*

A single unfamiliar word can open a door you didn't know was there.
So, I went looking.

What we call history now…
was once a warning.

Before the Term, There Was the Knowing

Long before there was language polished enough for textbooks, there was understanding. And communities carried those truths long before institutions admitted them.

Black communities didn't need studies or citations to know we were not safe. We watched bodies disappear. We noticed graves had been disturbed. We learned through experience, not paranoia, that hospitals were not always places of healing. That doctors did not always arrive with care in mind.

What later got dismissed as superstition or folklore was, in reality, observation. A record kept without pen or paper. Knowledge passed quietly... because speaking too loudly carried its own risks.

People warned each other.

Children were told not to wander at night.
Stories circulated - never casually, always with purpose.

The term *night doctor* didn't emerge from imagination. It emerged from necessity.

It was a name given to figures believed to operate under the cover of darkness, physicians, medical agents, men backed by institutions and authority, who took Black bodies for examination, experimentation, instruction, and harvesting. Bodies that were not volunteered. Bodies that were not returned whole. Bodies that often weren't returned at all.

This wasn't fear of medicine. It was a response to medicine as it was practiced.

Medical schools needed cadavers. Hospitals wanted data. Researchers chased discovery. And Black bodies, poor, enslaved, incarcerated, institutionalized, dehumanized, and devalued, were treated as... accessible. Available. Expendable.

Consent was rarely part of the equation. Humanity even less so.

So, communities did what communities have always done when systems fail them: they named the threat.

Night doctors became a warning label. A way to explain why mistrust lingered. Why survival required vigilance. Why care was often sought only as a last resort.

This knowledge didn't live in archives. It lived in bodies. In instincts. In the quiet tightening of a grip when a child strayed too far. In the collective memory that said: *something happens after dark*.

And that memory endured... because it had to.

A warning.

A whisper.

A truth learned the hard way.

Immortality Without Permission

The warnings whispered in the dark eventually showed up in the fluorescent light of hospitals.

Henrietta Lacks is often introduced as a lesson.
A cautionary tale.
A story we tell now as proof we've learned from the past.

But through the shadow of night doctors, her story stops being singular.
It becomes familiar.

Her cells were taken during treatment at Johns Hopkins in 1951, under conditions where consent was neither informed nor freely given.

No explanation.
No warning.
No option to refuse.

What followed was scientific immortality: cells that replicated endlessly, fueling breakthroughs in cancer research, virology, genetics, and medicine itself.

HeLa cells changed the world.
But progress built on silence is still theft.

Henrietta Lacks did not get to decide that.

For decades, her family didn't know her cells were still alive, circulating, multiplying, profiting institutions that never acknowledged her name.

When they did learn, it wasn't through outreach or accountability.
It came through discovery, confusion, and the slow realization that a piece of her life had been taken through omission and silence… and never returned.

This is where the language of progress gets slippery.

Because immortality sounds like honor.
Breakthroughs sound like justification.
And cures have a way of quieting the questions we don't want asked.

But strip the story down to its essentials, and it mirrors the old warnings:

A body accessed through deception or assumed compliance.
Knowledge extracted without informed permission.
Benefit flowing in one direction.

The only difference… lighting.

And maybe that's why it's easier to accept.

What happens in the dark feels secretive and distant.
What happens in plain sight…

requires a different kind of acknowledgment and accountability.

Night doctors didn't disappear.
They evolved.

They moved indoors.

They learned how to make consent sound official, even when refusal was never truly an option.

They put on credentials. Many already had them.

They learned how to make theft sound clinical.
Necessary. Inevitable.

And once the harm could be framed as an unfortunate oversight rather than an intentional practice, it became easier to forgive.

Easier to compartmentalize.

Easier to say *that was then*.

But this wasn't an isolated ethical lapse.
It was a continuation.

Henrietta Lacks didn't create mistrust of medicine in Black communities.
She confirmed it.

Her story didn't introduce a new injustice.
It pointed to an old one - rooted, repeated, and ignored.

And if that kind of violation could happen in the fluorescent light of a hospital, documented, normalized, defended, then the whispers about what happened in the dark begin to sound less like rumor...
and more like record.

Receipts: Proof Left in Plain Sight

Louisiana.

The nineteenth century bleeding into the twentieth.

Somewhere between curiosity and cruelty, heads were severed from Black bodies for research. Cadavers dismembered in the name of medical advancement. Stored. Cataloged. Labeled. Studied.

This wasn't metaphor. It was method.

In the 1870s, after Black patients died at Charity Hospital in New Orleans, many of them poor, many formerly enslaved, a physician removed their skulls and sent them to Germany.

Not for burial. For study.

Their skulls didn't just disappear... they were taken. Collected. Cataloged. Studied.

Turned into evidence for phrenology, a racist pseudoscience built on the lie that intelligence, morality, even human worth, could be measured by the shape of a skull.

They became specimens.

For more than a century, those skulls sat in a German university collection, anonymous, detached from families, stripped of context and dignity. Removed from community memory. Removed from humanity.

As reported by NPR in May 2025, it took until 2023 for the University of Leipzig to formally acknowledge that the remains had been acquired unethically.

What followed was not a reckoning, but a process. Slow. Administrative. Careful in a way the original act had never been.

In 2025, the remains of nineteen Black Americans were finally returned to New Orleans and laid to rest with a multi-faith memorial and a traditional jazz funeral... a gesture of dignity long overdue.

This return does not erase what happened.

For decades - elsewhere and everywhere - other remains stayed in university collections.

Heads.
Bones.

Bodies taken under coercion, omission, or manufactured consent.

Held in the name of knowledge.

Sometimes decades passed before anyone outside the institution knew they existed.
Sometimes the truth never surfaced at all.

And when recognition came, it rarely arrived as restitution.
More often, it came as ceremony.
As language.
As apology without consequence.

The structure is unmistakable.

Black bodies were treated as raw material.
As objects.
As property claimed under the banner of progress.

The same logic repeated in laboratories, hospitals, and medical schools.

Consent existed when it was convenient... on paper, not in practice.
Humanity was often absent.

Henrietta Lacks.
The Louisiana skulls.

Night doctors.

Frankenstein.

Different names.

Different decades.

Different settings.

The impulse was identical.

Take what is not yours.

And call it progress.

History shows the consequences. Families know them. Communities remember them.

And still, the systems that allowed these violations remain. Quieter now. More polished. More careful with language. Still insisting that the pursuit of knowledge justifies the theft of bodies, the erasure of identity, and the silencing of voices, even when permission was extracted through deception.

A warning.

A whisper.

A truth learned the hard way.

And the body carries what the record refuses to hold.

The Making of Monsters

To understand the mindset behind these violations, we have to look beyond history and into the stories we tell about creation and power.

Mary Shelley didn't write *Frankenstein* as a fantasy about monsters. She wrote it as a warning about men who believe themselves entitled to create without consequence.

Victor Frankenstein never asks permission. He doesn't pause to consider the origin of the bodies he collects or the ethics of their use.

He sees only potential, parts assembled for purpose, flesh reduced to material.

What mattered was the achievement. The proof that he could.

Sound familiar?

The horror of Frankenstein isn't the creature.

The creature is thoughtful, observant, emotionally aware. He learns language. He longs for connection. He understands rejection. He is, for all intents and purposes, human, and therefore inherits human qualities.

His violence comes later.

After abandonment. After being denied dignity. After being treated as an error instead of a being.

Through this lens, the true monster is the maker.

Victor creates life and immediately recoils from it. He refuses responsibility. He frames his horror as justified disgust rather than moral failure.

The creature becomes dangerous not because he exists, but because he is denied the most basic human need: recognition.

This is where the line between literature and history thins.

Night doctors, like Victor Frankenstein, operated under the belief that ambition outweighed consent. That the pursuit of knowledge justified the means.

Let me say that again...

The pursuit of knowledge justified the means.

That bodies, especially Black bodies, could be taken, studied, altered, and discarded in the name of progress.

Shelley captured, perhaps unintentionally, the psychology of medical entitlement:

- The belief that curiosity grants access.
- That brilliance absolves harm.
- That discovery erases debt.

Victor Frankenstein's laboratory was fictional.
The logic behind it was not.

Medical science has long depended on bodies rendered anonymous... stripped of names, families, and futures.

When those bodies belonged to the powerless, the ethical line blurred quickly.

When they belonged to Black people, it often disappeared altogether.

And just like in Shelley's novel, the aftermath was never owned.

The suffering created in pursuit of greatness was framed as unfortunate.
Incidental.
Necessary.

Responsibility was displaced - onto history, onto standards of the time, onto the very people who were harmed.

Read this way, *Frankenstein* feels less like gothic fiction and more like a confession written before anyone was ready to admit the truth.

The monster was never the body on the table.
The danger has always been the belief that some bodies exist for others to use.

It was the hand that believed it had the right to take.

What the Body Remembers

Bodies carry more than events... they carry how they were handled, how they were touched, whether consent was honored or manufactured, whether trust was met with care or quietly violated.

The body carries what no archive can fully contain: muscle, bone, blood, lineage, inheritance. Trauma lodges itself there, sometimes silently, sometimes erupting without warning. It settles into posture, breath, instinct. Into what feels safe… and what never quite does.

When we speak of night doctors, of Henrietta Lacks, of severed remains, the horror isn't only in the act. It's in the echo.

Bodies that were taken, studied, altered, and discarded did not forget. They are proof.

And the descendants of those bodies inherit the aftermath. What remains is mistrust, wariness, and a vigilance born not of imagination, but of survival.

This imprint is layered. It shows up in instinct, in hesitation before signing a form, in questions asked twice, in the pause before trusting a system that has not always been trustworthy. It lives in stories passed quietly between generations, in warnings about the dark, in the understanding that what is done to your body can ripple outward, touching lives not yet lived.

The body remembers what the mind sometimes cannot because survival often depends on it. That memory, unspoken and embodied, becomes its own form of continuation.

This is the inheritance of Black bodies in America: knowledge learned the hard way, vigilance encoded in flesh,
history etched in veins and bones, identity braided from trauma and resilience.

And still - the body is not only a vessel of harm. It is also a site of reclamation.

It can be a guide... a teacher, a map back to what was taken, what was denied, and what must now be named.

Naming becomes an act of refusal - the refusal to forget, to minimize, to allow dignity to remain deferred.

The body remembers...
and refuses erasure.

Choosing to Name It

Naming becomes power. Witness. Refusal.

We call them *night doctors* because silence was never enough. Whispered warnings, hushed stories, cautious glances - those were survival. Naming them aloud is reclamation. It is memory transformed into record. It is history refusing erasure.

To say *night doctors* is to insist: the harm happened, the bodies were taken, consent was manipulated, and trust was broken. And the legacy persists. It is a refusal to let progress be measured only by breakthroughs, discoveries, or profit.

Choosing to name it also honors survival. Families persisted, communities remembered, and the stories survived despite fear. Knowledge was safeguarded in whispers, in rituals, in embodied understanding. Naming becomes an act of respect for those who endured and for those who were never given the chance to refuse.

This is the threshold where memory becomes choice. Where inherited trauma is not only carried, but recognized, understood, and used to guide decisions, personal and collective.

The bodies may have been taken, the voices silenced, the histories buried... but naming restores something that cannot be confiscated: agency.

We end here not with arrival, but with intention. Memory has been honored. Now it has to be used.

And using it means facing what was actually done... fully and without looking away.

Once it's written down, it feels settled.

That doesn't make it complete.

The Record

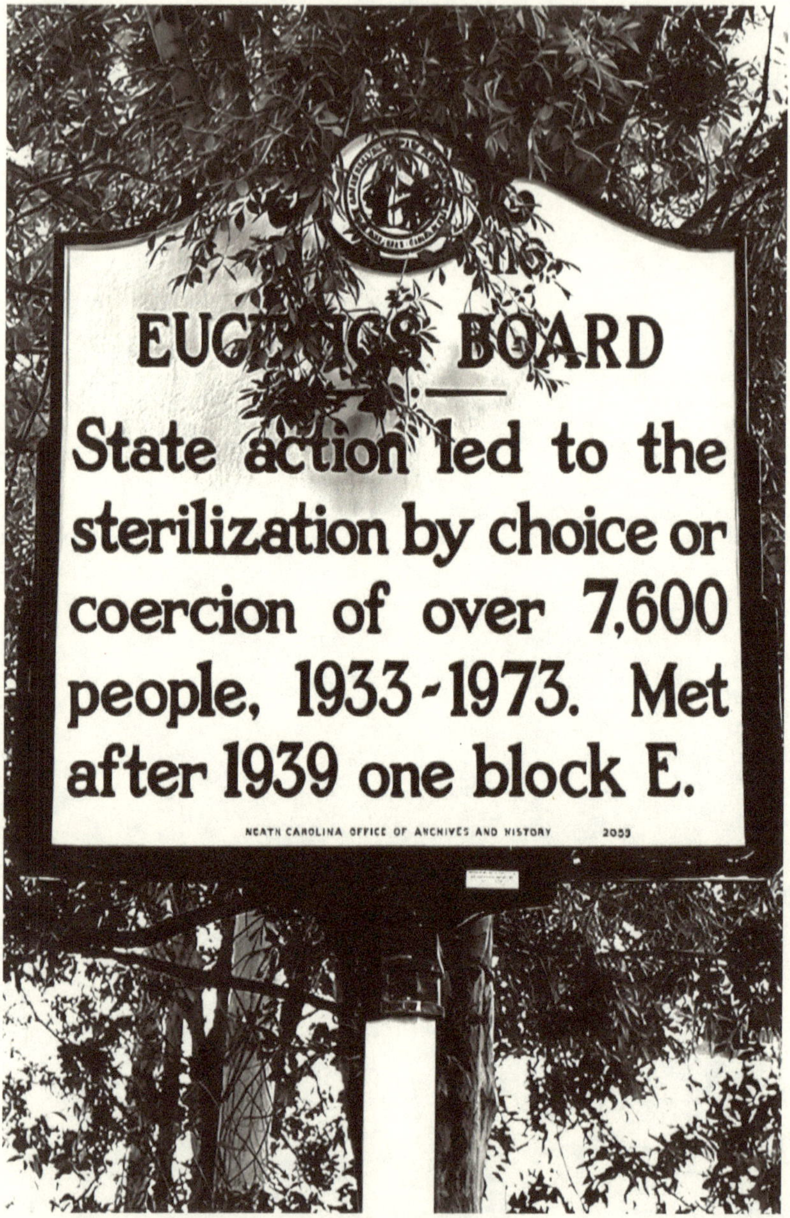

Historic Marker - Downtown Raleigh, NC - McDowell St + W Jones St

The Body Keeps Score

The body keeps score. So do we. Not just of what happened to us… but of what happened before us.

It's one thing to inherit blood type. Another to inherit a distrust so deep it shows up before you even sit down in the waiting room. Before the thermometer beeps. Before the gown opens in the back. Before the white coat enters.

Some of us already feel uneasy before a word is spoken.

That unease isn't paranoia.
It's history. Sometimes, it's inherited.

History doesn't disappear.
It settles into instinct.

I've seen versions of it my entire life.

Growing up, pain was rarely treated as an emergency. It was something to work through. Something to manage. Something that would eventually pass if you gave it enough time.

"It'll be alright."

"Put something on it."

"Give it a few days."

Those weren't just responses to discomfort. They were lessons. Lessons passed quietly from one generation to the next.

My grandmother spent years working in healthcare as a CNA. She cared for other people for a living, yet she still trusted old remedies, salves, and home treatments for many of her own ailments.

It wasn't that she rejected doctors. I remember going with her to appointments when I was young. Her physician, Dr. Salter Cochran, an older silver-haired Black man in a white coat, operated his practice out of a mauve-and-peach-colored house.

And just now, as I write this, I'm realizing the significance, and rarity, of her doctor being a Black man in the mid- to late 1970s. I never really thought about that until this moment.

The office was downstairs. He lived upstairs.

I remember sitting in the waiting room on these oversized brown leather sofas while she disappeared behind a door. The room always felt cold. The music always seemed strangely somber.

Even now, I can still see it. Hear it. Smell it.

But for all those visits, healthcare was never the center of her life. It was something you used when necessary. Something you turned to when the remedies stopped working.

My aunt taught me something different.

The day we realized something was seriously wrong wasn't the day she got sick. It was the day she could no longer hide how sick she had become.

I hadn't heard from her, and I had this eerie feeling. So, I asked a friend to check on her because she was closer, but I was on my way. What they found led to an ambulance ride and an immediate trip to intensive care. She was severely dehydrated. Her lips were white and peeling. Her body had been carrying far more than anyone knew.

It was then that we learned she had advanced AIDS.

And I distinctly remember the doctor telling me if you had waited one more day. And the idea of that was more than I could bear alone.

To this day, I can't tell you exactly why she carried that burden alone. Shame, I'm most certain, played a role. Privacy may have too. The lack of insurance absolutely did. Maybe all of them did.

What I do know is that she wasn't the first person to delay care because the path to receiving it felt too complicated, too expensive, too uncertain, or too exposing.

My mother sits somewhere between those worlds.

She goes to the doctor. She listens. She follows up.

But she's also looking for another answer. Another option. Another possibility. Something that might help without another prescription, another procedure, another specialist.

When she has appointments now, I try to go with her whenever I can. If I can't, I send my son. Not because she isn't capable of advocating for herself, but because somebody needs to hear the information. Somebody needs to ask questions. Somebody needs to fill in the gaps.

My mother has a habit of deciding what is and isn't important before she ever gets to the appointment. A fall that happened last week. A headache that lasted three days. A pain she has been quietly managing for months. To her, those details might seem unrelated. To a doctor trying to understand the full picture, they matter.

So one of us goes with her.

Not to speak for her.

To make sure the whole story gets told.

Then there's my uncle.

Lord have mercy.

If there is a conspiracy theory hiding in the room, he'll find it.

But underneath the skepticism is something more complicated. He's impatient as hell and he's a veteran. Years of navigating systems, paperwork, approvals, delays, and conflicting answers have shaped how he sees healthcare. What looks like distrust on the surface often feels more like exhaustion underneath. When every interaction requires another form, another call, another explanation, faith in the process becomes difficult to maintain.

And then there is me.

I would love to tell you that I stand outside all of this. That I learned from every example and always make the right decision.

I don't.

Living with arthritis while navigating periods of unemployment has forced me into calculations I never expected to make, again, at this stage of my life. You lose full-time employment and apply for assistance, only to be told you don't qualify because you make too much money in unemployment. Imagine that!

Your unemployment runs out and you're fortunate enough to get a part-time job. Still, you make too much money to qualify or to receive enough aid to meaningfully ease the burden. You don't qualify for programs that seem designed for people in exactly your situation.

After a while, you say the hell with it.

Because you don't know what you don't know and that's half the battle, right?

Meanwhile, your knees still hurt.

So sometimes you grit your teeth. You adjust. You endure. Not because the pain isn't real, but because there doesn't appear to be another option.

The fortunate part of my story is that I have nurse practitioners who know me. People who have knowledge, access and the willingness to help navigate systems often feel impossible to navigate alone. People who have built relationships with me over years. People who understand my circumstances beyond what appears on a chart.

Their care has often been the difference between navigating the system and giving up on it.

I never looked at my family's experiences as catalysts. But as this book has come together, I can see how each has informed the larger narrative.

My grandmother's remedies.

My aunt's silence.

My mother's caution.

My uncle's skepticism.

My own calculations.

Now I see them differently.

They are not identical stories, but each reveals the separate ways people learn to live with pain, uncertainty, cost, and distrust. Together, they speak a language shaped by access, experience, trust, survival, and history.

The body keeps score.

Families do too.

What do you call it when a system meant to heal
becomes one that harms?
When your DNA carries the echo of someone else's
blade?

For many of us, the answer isn't theoretical.
It's inherited.

This chapter isn't about mistakes. It's about people, communities, generations of bodies turned into battlegrounds - tested, silenced, controlled, erased.

Some names remain. Most do not.

But something remains with them... in whispered conversations, in chronic hesitation, in the quiet decision not to go back.

The stories survived... even when they told us to forget. Silence doesn't erase the truth; it simply forces it underground.

And nowhere is that buried history clearer than in the stories we were never meant to know.

Tuskegee - The Lie Was the Diagnosis

Officially, it was called *The Tuskegee Study of Untreated Syphilis in the Negro Male.* The title identified the subjects. The study itself revealed their worth in the eyes of the people running it.

Let that sit for a moment.

Language has always been one of the first tools of erasure.

What, exactly, made the "Negro male" such an attractive subject for decades of observation?

To understand the cruelty, you have to understand the worldview that made it possible.

Context matters.

The study began in 1932, in the thick of Jim Crow and the Great Depression - a time when Black people were openly deemed inferior, intellectually deficient, promiscuous, and unreliable when it came to healthcare. In other words: Expendable. Convenient. Targetable. The study didn't happen *despite* these beliefs - it happened *because* of them.

Syphilis, according to modern medicine, is a bacterial infection that is most often spread through sexual contact. It can lie dormant for years, quietly damaging the heart, brain, and nervous system before symptoms appear. By the 1940s, penicillin was a known, effective treatment.

In Macon County, Alabama, trust was the bait. Exploitation was the plan. Six hundred Black men signed up for what they believed was free healthcare. What they received instead was forty years of calculated harm.

Forty years is not a mistake. It's a commitment.

From 1932 to 1972, the U.S. Public Health Service tracked untreated syphilis in these men even after treatment existed. No informed consent. No real explanation. No intervention. Silence wasn't accidental... it was engineered.

The study involved 399 men with latent syphilis and 201 uninfected men used as a control group. All were poor. Many were sharecroppers, men with no leverage and even less protection.

Poverty didn't just make them eligible... it made them targetable.

The study hid behind the phrase "Bad Blood," a catch-all term that sounded familiar, folksy, and conveniently vague. It was language deliberately simplified for men researchers believed would be easier to mislead.

There was a prevailing presumption among researchers that syphilis affected Black men differently, that it caused cardiovascular damage more than neurological damage. This assumption was conveniently contrasted with prior research conducted on white men in Oslo, Norway.

And then came the unspoken logic: neurological damage impacts the brain. Intelligence. Cognition. And if Black men were already assumed to lack intelligence, why bother studying that part at all?

The lie wasn't just in the diagnosis... it was the belief that these men mattered less.

Pseudo-treatments followed. Mercury rubs, placebos, arsenic, painful spinal taps framed as "special procedures." The men were never told they had syphilis. Never warned they could infect their wives. Never told their children could be born with it. And when penicillin became widely available? It was deliberately withheld.

The betrayal rippled outward. Families were destroyed. Communities learned, slowly and painfully, that trust could be fatal.

Eunice Rivers, a Black nurse from the community, became the face of the study. She was skilled. Trusted. Respected. And she was the bridge the experiment relied on. Care and betrayal lived in the same hands. Her role remains complicated, contested, unresolved.

By the end of the study, only seventy-four of the 399 infected men were still alive. Twenty-eight died directly from syphilis. One hundred more died from related complications. Forty wives were infected. Nineteen children were born with congenital syphilis.

Tuskegee wasn't an anomaly. It was a blueprint.

The names change.
The design doesn't.

Henrietta Lacks - Taken Without Asking

Tuskegee denied care. Henrietta Lacks had care taken from her.

We've already met the night doctors - the ghosts who haunted Black imagination long before consent forms existed. Henrietta's story echoes an older fear, but in fluorescent light instead of darkness.

In 1951, Henrietta Lacks walked into Johns Hopkins Hospital alone, seeking treatment for cervical cancer. She was treated. She was not informed.

Without her knowledge or consent, cells from her tumor were taken during treatment. Those cells - later named

HeLa - did what no human cells had done before: they lived. They multiplied. Endlessly.

Her cells went on to change modern medicine - without her knowledge... without her consent. Polio vaccines. Cancer research. Gene mapping. Space research. Entire industries built on their replication.

Henrietta died months later.

Her family didn't know about her cells for decades.

No consent. No compensation. No acknowledgment.
And ultimately, no choice.

This wasn't a mistake. It was a decision.

The system didn't fail Henrietta. It functioned exactly as designed... extracting value while erasing the person it came from.

The theft was quiet. Surgical. Efficient.

There were no decades of observation, no mass casualties in a single county, just one woman, one moment, one decision that echoed forever.

Henrietta's story isn't about cells... it's about erasure. About invisibility. About how easily humanity can be edited out of progress. Because progress without consent has always had a familiar shape.

Her story wasn't an exception - it was part of a pattern that stretched far beyond one woman, one hospital, or one set of cells.

Different place.
Same assumption.

Puerto Rico - Pills, Promises, and Eugenics

She wasn't trying to join a movement - she was trying not to get pregnant again.

The clinic felt familiar. The promise was simple... birth control. Control over a life already stretched thin by poverty, obligation, and limited options. They called it modern medicine. Progress. Freedom.

What they didn't say was that she was stepping into an ideology that had already decided her value before she walked in.

Eugenics.

The belief that some people should reproduce - and others should not.

By the 1950s, eugenics no longer announced itself. It traded language. Lab coats replaced slogans. Control became "public health." Elimination became "population management."

Puerto Rico became a convenient testing ground. A U.S. territory, but not quite the United States. Brown women. Poor women. Women encouraged to trust clinics that promoted sterilization as routine - often framed as practical, even expected, after having children. *La operación.* Final. Permanent. Normalized.

When scientists needed human subjects to test the first oral contraceptive pill, they came to the island.

The pill was experimental. The dosage was far higher than what would later be approved. Women were not told this was a trial. Many were not fully informed of the risks. What consent was given was often incomplete, shaped by limited information and unequal power.

When they reported side effects, nausea, migraines, dizziness, blood clots, their complaints were dismissed. Their pain treated as background noise.

Three women died, and the work kept moving forward.

There were no serious investigations. No urgency. No accountability.

The pill worked. The data was collected. The formula was refined. The product was refined for the mainland, made safer for someone else.

And when researchers needed subjects even less likely to resist, they expanded into psychiatric institutions, where men and women labeled unfit were included in trials with even less oversight. Consent was irrelevant.

This was eugenics in practice.

Not shouted. Not branded. Methodical.

Who should reproduce? Who shouldn't? Who gets information?

Who gets managed?

The women lived with the aftermath long after the researchers left. Their bodies held on to what the reports erased.

Lateral Impact: When the Pattern Shows Itself

Tuskegee denied treatment. Henrietta's cells were taken. Puerto Rican women were coerced.

Different bodies. Different methods. The underlying belief never changed.

Medicine didn't malfunction. It performed exactly as designed when power went unchecked. These weren't isolated tragedies. They were coordinated outcomes of a system that decided whose bodies could be used, whose pain could be ignored, and whose futures could be altered in the name of progress.

Black men were observed. A Black woman was mined. Brown women were managed. Native women were sterilized. Disabled bodies were erased.

The bodies changed. The calculation did not.

This is why distrust didn't come from nowhere. It was taught. Passed down. Reinforced by lived experience.

The body retains what history tries to sanitize and what institutions try to forget.

This chapter isn't about rejecting medicine. It's about demanding accountability. About insisting that consent is not optional. That trust must be earned.

Healing requires truth. And truth requires reckoning.

What remains lives in the body whether institutions acknowledge it or not.

What followed was quieter, but no less deliberate.

Pain is persuasive.

When you're hurting, you don't interrogate the system... you negotiate with it. You trust the person with the pen, the badge, the letters after their name. You trust the system because relief is framed as its purpose. Because questioning feels like a luxury reserved for people who aren't in pain.

But pain has always been more than a symptom. In the wrong hands, it becomes leverage.

This chapter lives downstream from *Tested and Tossed*. No hidden trials. No midnight surgeries. No doctors sneaking data into ledgers. This time, the harm arrives neatly through paperwork, policies, prescriptions, and marketing decks polished to a shine.

Medicine didn't need to experiment anymore. It just needed to scale.

It learned how to monetize suffering cleanly, quietly, and for profit.

Another community. The cost was familiar.

Appalachia - When Relief Learned How to Lie

The pain was real - long before the pills arrived.

He'd been working the mines since he was nineteen. His father before him. His father's father, before that. It was just what you did, where he was from, where most people were from. The work was hard and the work was honest...

and eventually, the work took something from you.

That was understood. That was never the part anyone warned you about.

What nobody warned him about was the pill.

It lived in the backs of coal miners who bent themselves underground for decades. In the hands of factory workers whose grip never fully returned. In the knees of men who'd gone to war and came home to towns already disappearing.

This wasn't acute pain. It didn't resolve. It didn't heal.
It just... stayed.

By the mid-1990s, much of Appalachia was already in free fall. Coal jobs were drying up. Unions had lost their teeth. Hospitals were few and far between, and specialists were the kind of care you drove hours to reach - if you could afford the gas.

People weren't asking for miracles.

They were asking to stay upright.

That's when OxyContin entered the picture - not as a drug, but as a promise. Approved in 1995 and marketed aggressively soon after, it was framed as a modern solution for chronic pain.

Time-released.

Low addiction risk.

Safe for long-term use.

Doctors were trained to believe this and trained to reassure others. Patients were reassured. And in communities where one physician often served an entire town, trust moved fast and questions moved slowly.

What arrived didn't look dangerous. It looked clinical. Responsible. Covered by insurance.

Relief, finally, with paperwork to prove it.

Pharmaceutical companies knew exactly where they were.

Rural regions meant fewer eyes. Fewer regulators. Fewer journalists asking why prescription rates were climbing so fast.

And in towns built on labor, pain relief wasn't framed as indulgence. It was framed as duty.

This will help you work. Help you provide. Help you keep going.

What no one said out loud was that "going" had no end point, only escalation.

By the early 2000s, some Appalachian counties were receiving staggering volumes of opioid prescriptions, more pills than people, year after year.

When time-release mechanisms were defeated, crushed, or misused, companies knew.

They adjusted the messaging... not the distribution.

Addiction crept in quietly, then all at once.

Overdoses followed. Children were raised by grandparents or not raised at all. Towns hollowed out in a way that didn't make headlines because it didn't look dramatic. It just looked... tired.

And when the backlash finally came, when prescriptions were restricted and clinics shut down, the system didn't offer treatment. It offered distance.

Patients became addicts. Addicts became criminals. And the market simply shifted to heroin, then fentanyl.

Care exited the room the moment profit did.

This wasn't a mistake.
It was a model.

Appalachia wasn't chosen at random. It was chosen because pain was plentiful, oversight was thin, and the people mattered just enough to trust - but never enough to protect.

Different focus.
Same exploitation.

Native American Women - When Care Was Conditional

She goes to a clinic because she needs help.
That part matters.

She isn't reckless. She isn't careless. She isn't hiding.
She is seeking care in the place she's been told exists for exactly this reason. A clinic meant to serve her. A system meant to protect her health.

What she doesn't know, what she isn't told, is that help will come with terms.

Between the 1960s and 1970s, Native American women across the United States were sterilized at alarming rates through Indian Health Service facilities. Some were asked to sign consent forms they could not read. Some were told the procedure was reversible. Some were informed after the fact. Others were never meaningfully informed at all.

And many were given no choice, because choice disappears quickly when medical care is conditional.

This didn't begin with sterilization.

Long before reproductive control entered the exam room, Native bodies had already been targeted through another institution that claimed benevolence: the schools.

For decades, Native children were removed from their families and placed in government - and church-run boarding schools. They called it education. They called it civilization. They called it opportunity but in practice, it functioned as something else entirely.

What it was, in practice, was forced assimilation.

Languages were forbidden. Hair was cut. Names were replaced. Culture was treated as a disease to be cured. And for children who resisted - punishment followed. Often brutal. Often public. Always instructive.

The goal was never learning.
It was compliance.

I felt the full weight of this while watching *1923*. The series does not flinch. It portrays priests and nuns speaking openly about "stripping the soul" from Native girls. The violence is unashamed. Systematic. Framed as moral duty.

Those children are fictional.
The system that produced them was not.

Boarding schools trained the government and the public to see Native identity as a threat to be corrected, managed, erased. Once that logic took hold, the transition from cultural control to bodily control was not a leap. It was the next step.

By the time sterilizations became widespread, the groundwork had already been laid.

Native women were not vulnerable because they lacked intelligence or agency. They were vulnerable because access had been structurally narrowed to a single door. Indian Health Service facilities were often the only source of medical care available. And the Indian Health Service was - and remains - a federal agency.

Here is the quiet truth about jurisdiction.

While reservations are sovereign land in principle, medical authority rested with the federal government. Funding, staffing, oversight, and policy answered not to tribes, but to Washington. Sovereignty existed on paper. Healthcare existed in practice.

And practice has a way of overruling principle.

This was not the work of a few rogue doctors. It was a model - procedures performed during childbirth, tubal ligations carried out with little or no explanation, consent obtained under sedation or duress. Administrative language softened what was being done. Forms replaced conversations. Files replaced faces.

Eugenics did not arrive waving flags. It adapted. It learned how to speak softly. It learned how to look reasonable.

I recognized this again while watching *Yellowstone*. In a flashback scene, a young white man is warned that the white woman he is seeking care at a reservation clinic, will be sterilized if she is treated there. The receptionist does not whisper. She does not dramatize. She states it plainly, like an established fact.

That woman is fictional. She belongs to television.

The fear does not.

What the scene captures is the logic of the system: some bodies are allowed care only if they surrender choice. Fiction did not invent that truth. It reflected it.

For Native women, sterilization was not simply the loss of fertility. It was the disruption of lineage, the severing of continuity, the quiet erasure of future generations.

Children not born. Names not spoken. Stories never passed down.

This was never about individual decisions.

It was about managing populations.

What boarding schools tried to erase through culture, sterilization extended through biology.

What Appalachia reveals is how pain can be monetized. What this reveals is how existence itself can be regulated.

Different levers. Same entitlement.

The intent never really changed.

When care becomes conditional, consent becomes optional. And the body, always the body, preserves what policy tries to forget.

Ethnicity changed.
Practice did not.

Asian Communities - When Policy Made Pain Invisible

Imagine being stripped of property, rights, autonomy, and dignity by the very government that claims to protect you.

During World War II, the U.S. government forcibly removed Japanese Americans from their homes and placed them in internment camps across the country. Families arrived by bus and by train, carrying what little they could salvage of their lives.

But their bodies were not free.

Inside those camps, medical care existed - but it was inconsistent.
Neglectful more often than not. At times, it crossed into harm.

Resources were limited. Conditions were poor. And what should have been care often made things worse.

When the state labels your existence a logistical problem, the human disappears.

The body becomes something to manage, track, and control.

But this didn't start at the camp gates.

It started at the water.

Before internment, before the war, Asian immigrants arriving in the United States passed through Angel Island. It was an entry point.

It was also a checkpoint.

And waiting there was the U.S. Public Health Service, operating with a kind of authority that had very little to do with healing.

Bodies were inspected. Examined. Held for weeks, sometimes months.

They were not welcomed. They were evaluated.

Certain bodies were assumed to carry certain risks, and Asian immigrants were treated as probable carriers of disease in ways European arrivals were not.

The assumption came first. The examination followed.

That is medicine used as gatekeeping.
Care functioning as surveillance.
A white coat standing at the door, deciding who gets in.

By the time internment began, that framework was already in place.

Inside camps like Manzanar, Tule Lake, and Heart Mountain, medical systems were present. But they operated within a structure that had already defined these families as threats.

Detention, not dignity, shaped the conditions.

Facilities were inadequate. Resources were thin. Procedures were carried out in environments that would not have been accepted elsewhere.

And yet, that part of the story rarely appears in the way history is told.

We frame it as a civil liberties failure. A wartime decision. A moment of fear turned into policy.

All of that is true.

But it is also a story about the body -
and what happens when the system responsible for care
has already decided what that body represents.

Across the Pacific, during the same era, a different policy took shape.

In 1948, Japan enacted the Eugenic Protection Law.

Pause there for a moment.

1948.

Three years after Hiroshima. Three years after Nuremberg.

After the world had already seen what eugenics could become and said it would not happen again.

And yet, it did.

For decades, the law allowed for forced sterilizations.

Tens of thousands of procedures. Women were targeted most often. Disabled individuals, disproportionately. People labeled unfit by a system that quietly determined whose futures were worth protecting.

The law remained in place until 1996.

Not 1956.

Not even 1976.

1996.

A formal apology did not come until 2019. Compensation arrived with it.

Some survivors had already died waiting.

What stands out is not only the harm, but how easily it blended into the background.

There were no mass declarations and no public reckoning in real time... just policy, documentation, language that made the outcome sound administrative rather than irreversible.

Eugenics did not disappear after World War II. It adapted. It learned how to present itself differently.

Back in the United States, the damage moved in another direction.

This time, it did not arrive through detention or legislation.

It arrived as an idea.

The model minority myth.

The assumption that Asian communities are self-sufficient, resilient, and unlikely to struggle in ways that demand attention.

It sounds like praise.

In practice, it narrows what providers expect to see.

When a clinician enters the room already assuming the patient is stable, unlikely to be in crisis, unlikely to present with something unexpected - that assumption shapes the interaction.

What gets asked. What gets pursued. What is set aside because it does not fit the expectation.

The impact is subtle: a follow-up question not asked, a symptom noted but not investigated, a diagnosis that seems close enough to close the case.

The patient often senses that something is off.
But experience has taught them that pushing too hard can come with consequences.

So, they don't.

And the assumption remains intact.

Pain that is not clearly expressed is missed. Conditions that present differently are explained away. And the outcome is uncertainty, sometimes for far longer than it should be.

There is no headline. No singular moment that defines it. Just harm that accumulates over time.

What stands out is how differently this pattern moves compared to the other histories in this book.

There are no formal study groups here. No withheld treatments. No single moment that signals what is happening.

Just invisibility.

At the border, determining who was worthy of entry. Inside the camps, where the full scope never fully entered the historical record. In the clinic, where assumptions shape what care becomes.

When the state defines a group as a threat, the human is reduced. When culture defines a group as successful, their struggles are minimized.

Different mechanisms. Same erasure.

Across countries, across decades, across systems, the continuity remains.

Some bodies are managed, some are processed, and some are overlooked.

And no one is asked to answer for it.

The record tells us what was done.
It rarely tells us what was dismissed.

Or who was never fully seen in the first place.

The Thread That Never Breaks

These stories do not just mirror each other. They rhyme.

Pain. Profit. Policy. Pattern.

Appalachia. Native women. Asian communities. Different targets, different decades, different mechanisms, but the underlying logic remains remarkably consistent.

Identify vulnerability. Administer control under the guise of care. Hide harm behind policy, paperwork, or protection. Trust the system because the system asks for trust.

Race mattered. Class mattered. Disability mattered. Citizenship mattered.

But once a system learns to justify harm bureaucratically, malice is no longer required. Momentum becomes enough.

And the damage continues long after the policy, study, or institution has learned how to rename itself.

What We Dare to Call Care

Medicine did not lose its way. It followed incentives.

Communities paid the price, every. single. time.

This chapter is not about villains twirling mustaches. It is about systems, carefully calibrated, painfully efficient, willing to extract value from suffering without a scalpel, without a scream, and sometimes without anyone noticing.

Pain became a business model, and business was good.

Silence became compliance by design. Trust became collateral damage, predictable, measurable, and ignored.

And still, the body remembers.

The question now is not whether this happened. The question is whether we recognize it when it wears a different name, a different uniform, a different prescription, a different policy.

White Bodies, White Data

What We Didn't Know We Were Missing

I've spent a fair amount of time in waiting rooms.

Waiting rooms with the same magazines nobody reads. The same diagrams on the wall, bodies cross-sectioned, labeled, explained.

I never thought much about those diagrams, but I did think about the magazines and how they didn't cater to me or people who looked like me.

But they were... there. Part of the furniture. Something to keep you entertained while you wait.

And the diagrams were just a part of medicine, neutral, official, the way things were supposed to look.

Isn't it funny how the magazines bothered me, but it never occurred to me, not once, that I had never seen myself in any of the diagrams?

Not really.

Not until someone else pointed it out.

Sometime after the initial COVID panic had settled, but in the midst of the national reckoning sparked by the murder of George Floyd, conversations about culture, equity, and who gets counted stopped being abstract and started colliding with real consequence.

It was during that stretch that an image surfaced on LinkedIn.

It wasn't sensational or loud, and it didn't arrive wrapped in explanation.

It was a medical illustration, a Black fetus in utero, created by Chidiebere Ibe.

And it stopped me like everyone else.

Its intent was not shock or spectacle, but revelation: an absence most people never realized was there.

The response wasn't framed around novelty. It was framed around recognition. We didn't know what we were missing because we had never seen it.

When a body isn't represented, it isn't just unseen. It's misunderstood.

And that misunderstanding, in medicine, has consequence.

That refrain surfaced again and again in the responses, and it mattered. It named a failure that had gone largely unexamined in medical spaces.

Representation, in this context, wasn't about affirmation or inclusion as ideology.

It was about baseline - what had quietly been established as normal... and what had been excluded without question.

We often hear the phrase: *If you don't see yourself, how can you envision yourself?*

In medicine, that question cuts deeper.

This isn't about imagination.

It's about instruction.

Medical illustrations are not neutral. They are not decorative. They are instructional tools. They train the eye. They shape expectation. They teach students what to recognize before they ever touch a patient. Long before a diagnosis is made, the visual record has already done its work.

Medical education trains clinicians to recognize patterns, but only within a limited visual and cultural frame. When that frame excludes entire populations, error becomes predictable.

This isn't about bedside manner or individual bias. It's about repetition. When nearly every diagram, chart, and image reflects the same body, that body becomes the reference point. Everything else is measured against it. Symptoms that don't match the visual baseline are labeled atypical. Conditions that present differently are more easily missed. Pain that doesn't look familiar is more readily minimized.

In that environment, misdiagnosis is not an anomaly.
It is an outcome.

What that illustration exposed wasn't just absence. It exposed how thoroughly that absence had been normalized. For decades, medical journals, textbooks, and training materials centered one body as standard. Others appeared rarely, if at all, sometimes reduced to side notes, sometimes framed only in pathology, often omitted entirely.

And we absorbed that.

Implicitly and consistently, the message was clear: our bodies did not require the same level of documentation. Our differences did not demand visual specificity. Our presence was not necessary for medical understanding to be considered complete.

That wasn't accidental.
That was instructional.

The moment that image appeared, representation stopped being a cultural argument and became a clinical one. Because suddenly the question wasn't *why does this matter?* - it was *how did we ever think it didn't?*

Disease does not present the same way across all skin tones. Symptoms do not manifest identically across bodies shaped by different genetics, environments, and histories. When the white body is treated as universal, everyone else becomes deviation - and deviation is where care falters.

This is how invisibility shows up in education.

Not through hostility, but through omission. Not through refusal, but through normalization.

And once omission is normalized, its consequences compound: misdiagnosis, delayed treatment, dismissed concerns. All layered atop existing assumptions about pain tolerance, credibility, and worth - assumptions that have long followed people of color into exam rooms.
The drawing didn't create awareness.
It exposed a void.

And it made the absence impossible to ignore:

You cannot diagnose what you were

never taught to see.

What Carries Forward

More than we were told.

For most of my life, I was convinced I was part Irish or German.

I have no idea where I got that from.

As a preteen, I remember sitting in my grandparents' house on my father's side, staring at an old black-and-white photograph hanging on the wall. The person in the picture looked White to me, and for whatever reason I decided that must mean Irish or German ancestry was hiding somewhere in our family tree.

Like a lot of Black Americans, I was equally convinced there was Native American ancestry in the mix. My father and his parents had what people used to call "good hair." I didn't inherit it, but I figured if it was part of them, then surely some of it had to be part of me.

Those assumptions sat quietly in the background for years.

Meanwhile, on my mother's side of the family, at reunions, photographs started appearing.

Pictures of my great-great-grandmother. Relatives I had never seen and barely heard mentioned before. Faces attached to names I had only heard mentioned in passing.

And then came Henry Louis Gates and his partnership with PBS.

Watching *Finding Your Roots* felt like watching people recover pieces of themselves. I was fascinated by what researchers could uncover, but I was equally fascinated by where the trail stopped. Again and again, Black families encountered the same wall.

Slavery.

Everyone else seemed able to keep going - in many cases for centuries.

We couldn't.

That realization stayed with me.

Eventually I joined Ancestry.com and submitted my DNA.

When the results came back and showed a small percentage of Scottish ancestry, I felt absurdly validated.

I knew it.

Black Irish!

At least that's what I told myself.

But the percentages turned out to be the least interesting part.

The records were where things became real.

Leaves started appearing. Documents surfaced. Branches of the family tree began unfolding. Stories I half remembered from childhood suddenly had names attached to them. Conversations I wasn't supposed to be listening to. The grown folks' business I absorbed while pretending to be quiet.

For the first time, pieces that had always existed separately began connecting to one another. The deeper I looked, the more I realized the gaps had not appeared by accident. Some were born of silence. Others of shame. Others of history. Some simply because information had been lost, softened, or never passed down at all.

Many of the things I found myself wanting to know had never been told in the first place... at least not to me. Truth be told, there was a time when I couldn't have cared less.

There is a limit to what family history can give us.
It relies on memory - on what was spoken, what was explained, and what survived long enough to be passed down intact. But as documents close and stories thin, that line breaks. What remains is often partial, simplified, or unresolved. Not because families failed to preserve it, but because they were never given the full story to begin with.

At that point, knowing where you come from becomes more than curiosity.
It becomes corrective.

Heritage, and the biological record carried in our DNA, offers continuity where paperwork stops. It does not replace family history; it fills in what history could not hold. It carries information that was never explained, never written down, or never trusted to survive beyond the moment it was recorded.

This is not about prediction or certainty.
It is about context.

When stories are incomplete, what was never explained still matters.
When records are closed, lineage remains open.

Knowing one's genetic and ancestral makeup isn't about rewriting the past - it's about recovering what was lost in transmission.

And when the gaps are inherited...
so is the responsibility to understand them.

What becomes clear, once paperwork reaches its limit, is that silence does not mean absence. It means the record stopped short. Information continued to exist elsewhere... in bodies, bloodlines, and inheritances that did not require explanation to survive.

Family history depends on transmission. Stories must be told fully and accurately enough to endure repetition. But when stories fracture, when they are shortened, softened, avoided, or never spoken at all, continuity does not disappear. It simply moves.

This is where heritage begins to matter differently.

Not as nostalgia.

Not as proof.

But as record.

DNA answers a different question. Where paperwork documents outcomes and memory preserves fragments, DNA carries what was never filtered through comfort, language, or permission. It holds information that survived whether it was acknowledged, understood, or explained.

That matters when the story breaks.

Names endure.
Relationships survive.
Context erodes.

Heritage persists anyway.

Not because it is remembered.
Because it was carried forward.

This is not about uncovering a dramatic truth.

It is about restoring dimension.

Knowing one's genetic and ancestral makeup matters not for its ability to predict outcomes, but for what it restores. It adds texture where records have flattened experience and fills the negative space left by documents designed to close rather than carry forward.

What DNA offers, in this context, is not certainty.

It offers orientation.

For me, this understanding didn't arrive as a revelation. There was no single result that rearranged my sense of self, no ancestral discovery that demanded redefinition.

If anything, I was kind of just like, "oh," unsurprised mostly, with one quiet exception.

More European DNA than I might have expected... Irish.

No shock. No grief. But something much quieter.

It confirmed what history had already suggested, we are more than we appear.

Not enough to destabilize my identity. But certainly, enough to make silence feel less like absence... and more like protection, but from what?

Being seen too clearly.
Or perhaps, not clearly at all.

Heritage is not only about what we know.

It is also about what others assume when they look at us, and what those assumptions allow or deny.

History offers many examples where "passing" was not deception, but survival.

Where proximity to whiteness afforded safety, access, or mobility, often at the cost of erasure.

That cost does not end with the individual.

"Passing" does not only obscure identity; it interrupts transmission. Children inherit bodies without context, features without explanation, histories that were intentionally withheld or quietly set aside. They move through the world, read one way while carrying something else entirely, including medical, genetic, and cultural realities they were never taught to name.

I think about this not as theory, but as possibility.

A child light enough to "pass" may never be told the full story - not out of malice, but out of habit, fear, or the belief that silence is protection. They learn how to move safely. They learn which questions not to ask. They inherit access but not always understanding.

And in that silence, a vital part of who they are is lost.

Medical systems do not read us the way families do.
They can't.

Families carry context where medicine relies on what it can see. Medical systems rely on appearance, shorthand, and assumption as much as they rely on charts.

Flatten the identity. Obscure or simplify the heritage. And care follows.

Not intentionally.
Procedurally.

This is where knowing what carries forward matters.

DNA doesn't tell us who we are.
It complicates what the world thinks it sees.

It restores context where visibility has overwritten truth.
It offers a counterweight to assumption.

For those who "pass", and for those who come after them, heritage becomes less about discovery and more about reclamation. A way of ensuring that what survives is not only what was safe to show, but what was true.

What carries forward is not always dramatic.
Sometimes it is quiet.
Sometimes it is simply there.

And sometimes, recognizing it is enough to change how we see what has always been with us, waiting beyond paperwork, beyond assumption, beyond what we were told.

Diagnosis & Discovery

What We Don't Know Can Kill Us

My Story, My Body

I remember sitting in my doctor's office, talking with my doctor, who is of Asian descent, talking about turning forty-nine and the changes that come with it. It sounds ominous, but let's be honest… it kind of is.

This time, the conversation was specific.

Colon cancer.

She told me to schedule a colonoscopy. I wasn't fifty, the traditional benchmark, so I asked why.

Updated data showed that African Americans are more susceptible to developing polyps at younger ages and at higher rates, increasing the risk of colon cancer if those polyps go undetected.

Her message was direct: don't wait.

So, I didn't.

That moment stayed with me, not for its alarm, but for its precision. It was care informed by data that actually included people who look like me.

That distinction matters… especially because the person delivering that care didn't look like me but still understood what the data required.

That memory takes me back to an earlier chapter of my life, when I was much younger, dealing with irregular cycles.

At the time, I preferred a male physician. My reasoning was shallow and unexamined. Why would I want another woman poking around in my nether regions?

I was naive. And honestly, afraid of the implication… I know.

During one visit, I had a particularly uncomfortable conversation. I tried to explain what was happening with my body during intercourse. His responses were off, dismissive, disconnected from what I was actually trying to explain.

Thankfully, nothing overtly traumatic happened, and that matters. This wasn't malpractice. It was misalignment.

After my son was born in 1992, I switched to a female OB-GYN. The difference wasn't dramatic, but it was meaningful. The questions changed. The listening changed. The assumptions shifted.

What those experiences taught me, long before I could articulate it, was that identity shapes care. Not emotionally. Practically.

Who we are affects how we're heard, how our symptoms are interpreted, and how quickly concern is taken seriously.

A Chance Meeting - Or Something Else

One day, while driving Lyft, I picked up a woman I initially read as white. As we talked, she told me she identified as multicultural - and she said it with pride, no hesitation.

At one point, she reached her hand between the seats.

"What do you see?" she asked.

I noticed discoloration. Purple blotches. Pale patches running along her fingers. Nail beds slightly off. I hesitated, then guessed wrong.

She corrected me.

"It's vitiligo."

She told me about a doctor's visit. She'd gone in for something unrelated, and midway through the exam, the physician stopped.

"What's that on your hands?"

"I don't know," she said.

"You're not supposed to have that," he replied.

Only about six percent of white people develop vitiligo, he explained. He assumed she was white, because that's how she presented, how she identified, and how he read her. So, a DNA test was ordered.

The results came back: Irish. Scottish. Egyptian.

That's when it became clear - the issue wasn't rarity... it was that the doctor had already decided what her body was allowed to be.

"You know Egypt is in Africa, right?" she said, smiling - not to educate, but to connect the dots between her newly identified heritage... geography, ancestry, and what her diagnosis had been trying to say.

Her condition wasn't rare.
It was misread.

That moment stayed with me because it exposed the real problem: medical interpretation too often leans on visual and cultural shortcuts. Her body had been telling the truth the entire time.

The assumption was the error.

When the Baseline Is Wrong

That conversation reminded me of an episode of Grey's Anatomy - Season 17, Episode 4.

In it, a physician treats an Asian patient but relies on diagnostic norms built around white patient populations. He skips a broader scan, settles on what seems obvious, and nearly misses a condition that is far more common in patients of Asian descent: right-sided diverticulitis.

The mistake isn't ignorance. It's default.

What corrects the course isn't advanced technology... it's cultural and clinical context, brought in by another physician who recognizes what the baseline failed to account for. That oversight could have had severe consequences.

During the debrief, Dr. Bailey delivers the line that matters:

"Equal treatment isn't the same as equitable treatment."

That distinction isn't philosophical.
It's clinical.

Cultural identity isn't just how we see ourselves. It's how the world sees us - and how our bodies carry truths that paperwork doesn't.

Treating everyone the same assumes the baseline is universal.

It isn't.

Bodies differ. Disease presents differently. Risk profiles shift across ancestry, environment, and history. When those differences are ignored in the name of neutrality, care becomes uneven - and sometimes dangerous.

Sickle-Cell Trait

I have a friend; we'll call him Liam.

Liam is white - he's white-white... at least in how the world would read him. Freckled. Strawberry blonde. Small-town white.

The kind of white that has likely never had to interrogate his identity.

Liam has the sickle-cell trait.

Yes... you read that correctly.

It caught me off guard.

Because as far as I understood it, sickle cell lived in one place, one community...

the Black community.

That framing is incomplete, but powerful. And it shapes expectations.

And just like that... my understanding shifted.

"Well..." I said, shaking my head, "welcome to the cookout."

He laughed. "Thank you."

We moved on.

But that moment stayed with me.

And as I've alluded... moments like that aren't random.

They're revealing.

Sickle cell trait doesn't care how someone identifies or how they're perceived.

It follows lineage.

Not labels.

The mutation is a biological adaptation, in part, to malaria, rooted in regions where the trait once offered protection.

But it doesn't belong to just one group.

It shows up across multiple regions, the Mediterranean, the Middle East, parts of India, Latin America, the Caribbean, threads of history, migration, survival, and mixing...

that don't always present themselves neatly in family stories.

Biology doesn't move the way assumptions do.

Fast forward a few months later, as I'm building this book, I reach out to Liam and ask if he'd be part of it.

He says yes.

So here we are.

Liam's Story

Liam's story starts with the Coast Guard.

But in a way...

it almost ends there too.

He didn't even make it out of MEPS.

Not because he couldn't.

Not because he changed his mind.

But because of a detail buried quietly in his blood -

unspoken, unremembered...

stopped him before he even began.

On the second day of processing, there's an exercise in humility.

Stripped down to underwear... a room full of men moving through drills that feel equal parts routine and exposure.

Duck walks. Vision tests. Hearing tests. Hours of waiting. Standing. Sitting. Proving yourself.

Now in front of the doctor, she flips through his file...

casually.

Then pauses.

"Oh… that's interesting. Did you know you have sickle cell trait?"

He didn't.

And just like that…

everything shifted.

He wasn't sick. He wasn't dying. But he wasn't cleared to move forward either.

Sickle cell trait isn't the disease.

That distinction matters.

The disease, sickle cell, happens when both parents pass the gene. That's where the pain lives… where blood cells harden, bend, struggle to move the way they should.

The trait?

One gene. Often silent.

Most people live their entire lives without ever knowing. Unless someone goes looking.

"You'll need another test," she says. "Immediately."

There are numbers attached. Percentages. Cutoffs. Timelines.

A quiet calculation about whether his body, under pressure, under stress, under conditions most people never experience, would cooperate or become a liability.

He takes the test. It takes time.

But life doesn't pause just because a finding surfaces. He gets a job. Signs a lease. Builds something stable while the system decides whether he fits inside it.

At home, there weren't many answers.
Maybe his parents were told. Maybe they forgot. Maybe it never felt important enough to hold onto.

Either way... here it was.
Uninvited. Unexplained. True.

Months later, Liam hears from his recruiter.

You're cleared - when can you ship out?

But by then... his life had already shifted.

Now, at 24, he's starting to look. Not urgently. Not out of fear.
But from a quieter place: curiosity.

He told me this hadn't impacted him.
And maybe, by traditional measures... he's right.

No hospital visits, no pain crisis, no daily reminders.

It hadn't asked anything of him.

But impact doesn't always show up loudly.

It showed up in a room. In a chair. Across from a doctor flipping through paperwork.

A pause. A question.

It showed up at the exact moment his life was trying to move forward.

Just like that... a piece of his inheritance he never imagined had enough weight to slow everything down.

Not forever.
But long enough to change direction.

That's where this lives.
In that in-between space.

Not sick. Not insignificant.
Maybe hidden. Maybe forgotten. But never gone.

It does not ask for attention.
It waits for it.

And if you don't know to speak it... if no one knows to ask...
it disappears.

Until it doesn't.

Because a truth can live in your body for years, quiet, unclaimed, unconsidered, and still powerful enough to interrupt your life the moment someone else decides it matters.

It didn't change who he is.
But it introduced a possibility:

That who we think we are and what lives in us aren't always the same.

And that gap...
that's where the real story begins.

When the Signal is Missed

There are conditions we think we understand. Not because we've studied them in depth... but because we've been told where they belong. Who they affect. What they look like. When they show up.

That framework becomes a kind of shortcut -
a way for both patients and providers to move quickly through uncertainty.

Until something doesn't fit.

Hydrocephalus is one of those conditions, often explained simply: an abnormal buildup of fluid in the brain. Pressure that can affect development, function, and survival.

It can be identified before birth… sometimes as early as a routine ultrasound.

From there, the path turns clinical: monitoring, imaging, specialists, decisions.

But like many conditions tied to development and genetics…
the why isn't always clear.

Sometimes it's structural. Sometimes infection.
Sometimes genetic factors not yet fully understood.

And sometimes… it appears without a clear story attached.

That's where expectation quietly steps in.

When a condition is more commonly associated with certain populations… it begins to shape how we look for it. How we explain it. How far we investigate once it's found.

If a trait is considered rare in a particular group… it gets treated as an exception. An outlier. Something that just happened.

But "just happened" is rarely the full story.

Especially when genetics are involved.
Especially when ancestry is incomplete… or unknown…
or misunderstood.

The body doesn't rely on what we've been told about ourselves.
It responds to what's actually there.

And sometimes...
what's there hasn't been named yet.

BeBe's Story

There are moments when everything shifts... and no one tells you that it has.

BeBe was about twenty weeks pregnant when they saw it.
An ultrasound. A pause.
Then a quiet redirect: *we need you to go to Durham.*

That's how it starts sometimes.
Not with urgency, but with a change in tone.

More scans. More eyes.
And then the word:

Hydrocephalus.
Fluid on the brain.

They said it plainly. Clinically.
As if naming it explained it.

It wasn't.

She asked what caused it.

They said it was genetic.

And just like that... the ground shifted.

There's a particular kind of disorientation that comes with being told a condition is genetic... when you have no framework for what that means. No history. No warning. No context to reach back into and say - *oh... this runs in the family.*

As far as she knew... it didn't.

And yet, there it was.

They gave her options.

Termination being one.

She didn't take it.

That decision wasn't wrapped in theory or statistics - it was immediate. Grounded. Certain.

So, she carried.

And she waited.

And she lived inside the space between what they said would happen... and what actually did.

Doctors told her what her daughter wouldn't be able to do.

She wouldn't cry. Wouldn't hear. Wouldn't function the way a "normal" baby should.

A list of limitations... delivered before the child even arrived.

But when Cheyenne was born...

She cried.

She ate.

She responded.

Not perfectly. Not predictably.

But enough to disrupt everything they thought they knew.

And in hospice care, even the nurse questioned it:

Why is this baby here?

Because sometimes... prognosis speaks too soon.

Her daughter lived.

Not long... but she lived.

She lived, but not in the way they expected.

Cheyenne was born in December.

She passed in January.

And in that short window, she did what no data could predict.

She existed beyond expectation.

It would have been easy to leave the story there. To file it under grief. Under loss. Under "one of those things."

But BeBe didn't.

The word *genetic* never sat right.

Later, during another pregnancy, they tested.

Not just her.

Him.

The father.

And that's when the missing piece surfaced.

He was a carrier.

Not visibly. Not obviously.

Nothing that would have raised a flag in everyday life...

not even in his other children.

But somewhere in his lineage... it lived.

Quiet. Unnamed. Unclaimed.

And when it met BeBe's body -

it showed up... exactly as it was always going to.

Here's where the story shifts.

Hydrocephalus isn't screened for differently based on race.

It's found the same way it's always found: when something on an ultrasound doesn't look right.

But what happens next, how it's explained, how deeply it's investigated… that's where expectation can quietly step in.

Because BeBe and her partner are Black, this wasn't a condition anyone expected to see. No one was looking for it.
And in this context, it's more commonly associated, in medical understanding, with populations that didn't look like them.

That mattered.

Not in theory.
In expectation.

Because when a diagnosis isn't expected… it often isn't looked for.
And when it's not looked for… it isn't explained.

So, what do you do with that?

With a diagnosis that arrives before the story?
With ancestry that exists - but was never spoken aloud?
With a loss shaped, in part, by an unspoken inheritance?

You sit with it.
Or… you ask different questions.

BeBe chose something simpler.

She didn't chase it backward. Didn't unravel the lineage. Didn't try to reconstruct what history failed to record.

"It was what it was," she said.
"God's plan."

And as I sat with her... it was clear. That was enough.

But for the rest of us...
it raises harder questions.

What else is sitting in our bodies... waiting for the right conditions to reveal itself?

What else has been carried forward - not through stories... but through silence?

This wasn't just about a diagnosis.

It was about inheritance without awareness.
A history that didn't announce itself...
until it had to.

And by then,
it was already here.

The pattern didn't end.

It learned how to look different.

What Discovery Really Means

We like to believe medicine is objective. That it operates above culture. That data speaks for itself.

It doesn't.

Data is collected from bodies deemed worthy of study. Patterns are built from what is seen repeatedly. When the baseline is narrow, discovery follows suit.

What we don't know can kill us, not because the information doesn't exist, but because it was never prioritized, never visualized, never taught.

Discovery doesn't begin with answers.
It begins when we stop assuming the baseline tells the whole story.

And until medicine learns to see bodies fully, not just uniformly, diagnosis will continue to fail the very people who need it most.

Modern Echoes

Distrust doesn't come out of nowhere.
It has a memory.

For Black communities, it isn't paranoia. It's pattern recognition, a muscle built over generations, flexed every time medicine arrives with good intentions and a paper-thin explanation. Every time urgency is paired with silence. Every time "trust us" replaces transparency.

So, when COVID came, it didn't arrive alone.
It came carrying ghosts.

In early 2020, uncertainty moved faster than the virus itself. Guidance shifted constantly. Masks were required... until they weren't. The virus wasn't airborne... until it was. Information lagged behind reality, and clarity was always one step late. Hospitals filled. Hallways overflowed. The death toll rose in numbers that stopped feeling real.

For Black communities, this chaos felt familiar.

Not because the virus was known. Because the response was.

Confusion layered on top of history. Messaging changed without context. Decisions were made without explanation. Authority spoke quickly and corrected itself later, expecting trust to stretch indefinitely.

And then the vaccines came.

Community conversations asked the question: *Should I get vaccinated?* Public conversation framed the moment with their own question: *Why are people of color so hesitant?* The framing itself revealed the problem.

I remember a conversation with a coworker early in the rollout. She was white, and that matters - because the question she asked explained everything. She wanted to know why "we" were so reluctant to get vaccinated.

I paused. This wasn't confrontation. It was correction.

I explained the history. The legacy of medical experimentation. The long record of neglect followed by sudden urgency. I suggested she watch *Miss Evers' Boys*. Later, she came back to me and said she had no idea.

And I believe her.

There is no standard curriculum that teaches this history. No required training that connects Tuskegee to present-day clinical trial recruitment. No widely taught framework that explains why distrust might be rational rather than reactionary.

But lack of exposure doesn't negate impact.

Tuskegee didn't need to be explained to Black communities. Its shadow was already there - in kitchen table conversations, in church parking lots, in group texts, in the pause before rolling up a sleeve. Hesitation wasn't about rejecting science. It was about interrogating intent.

Speed didn't help.

For decades, communities of color experienced delayed care, underfunded hospitals, and poorer outcomes. Then suddenly, those same communities were prioritized without an equally urgent effort to repair trust. The question wasn't irrational:

If we were invisible before, why are we essential now?

Misinformation rushed into the gap where transparency should have been. Social media amplified fear, becoming both a megaphone and minefield... sometimes irresponsibly, sometimes because the claims weren't entirely implausible given history. When harm has been unevenly distributed, probability feels personal.

Clinical trials hovered in the background of these conversations. Different names. Softer language. Ethics boards and consent forms thick enough to intimidate. Participation framed as voluntary. Safeguards emphasized.

And yet the question lingered: *Who is this really for?*

Consent exists on paper. Understanding does not always follow. Side effects are discussed, but often minimized:

framed as rare, temporary, manageable. For communities that have historically borne the weight of those "rare" outcomes, reassurance doesn't land the same way.

Representation in trials is measured numerically - boxes checked, percentages met - but inclusion on paper does not guarantee protection in practice. Being present in data does not mean being understood. Participation does not ensure benefit.

For many Black Americans, clinical trials don't feel neutral. They feel transactional. Extractive. The body is welcomed; the voice not so much.

So, when people were asked, once again, to trust the process, the request did not arrive in a vacuum. It landed on a history of unanswered questions, of studies celebrated for outcomes while consequences were quietly absorbed, and of progress measured broadly while individual harm was treated as collateral.

This is the modern echo.

The decision to vaccinate wasn't singular. It was negotiated - between fear and responsibility, between personal safety and collective survival, between knowing the cost of participation and the cost of refusal.

Some chose vaccination immediately. Others waited.
Some never did. None of those choices were casual. What

was labeled "hesitancy" was often grief wearing caution. Memory wearing vigilance.

Modern distrust is not a rejection of progress.

It is an insistence on accountability.

And until healthcare systems reckon fully with their histories - not just acknowledging them, but repairing the damage they caused - distrust will continue to echo...

because the consequences never disappear.

And in this context, that is not the problem.

It is the warning.

The pattern doesn't end.

It adapts.

It refines itself.

It learns how to look different… while doing the same thing.

And it leaves its mark on everything - especially the symbols we stopped questioning.

More Than A Design Choice: The Warning We Ignored

The symbol was never meant to reassure us -
but to remind us that healing, mishandled, becomes harm.

By the time I finished writing this book, I had spent more time thinking about medicine than I ever expected to.

Not the medicine of today, but the throughlines in the medicine of yesterday. The waiting rooms. The clipboards. The forms that assumed you knew things you were never told. My body. Carrying a history no chart was ever designed to hold.

And then I looked at the cover.

This chapter was not part of the original plan.

It arrived after the cover was finished - after the symbolism had been chosen... placed... approved. The visual felt honest. Complete. Rooted. Intentional.

And yet, one element kept pulling my attention back to it.
Not loudly. Not insistently.
Just enough to make ignoring it feel careless.

The medical symbol on the back cover.

It wasn't dominant. It wasn't meant to be a focal point. But the longer I sat with it, the more it refused to remain just a design choice.

What I initially treated as aesthetic - a quiet part of the broader story - began to feel like an unanswered question... one I wasn't meant to overlook.

Why this symbol?

Why the snakes?

What's the relevance?

And more specifically...

Why does it sit at the center of modern medicine?

What started as a visual decision became an internal interrogation.

The image is familiar.

The symbol - two snakes wrapped around a staff - has been so normalized that most of us no longer notice it. It appears on hospital walls, prescription pads, ambulances, and insurance portals.

It signals authority. Expertise. Care.

We're not taught to question it.
We accept it the way we've been taught to accept so much of medicine: without interrogation.

But symbols don't become permanent by accident. They become permanent because no one challenges what they've come to represent.

The earliest version of this symbol was different.

One snake. Not two.

The Rod of Asclepius.

It wasn't designed to comfort. It was meant to reflect the truth about healing: Balance. Precision. Restraint.

The understanding that the same force capable of healing could just as easily harm… if mishandled.

That distinction mattered.

Because the snake was never meant to reassure.

It was meant to warn.

Somewhere along the way, the image shifted.

One became two.

The caduceus - associated not with healing, but with Hermes.

A messenger. A guide of travelers. A protector of merchants… and thieves alike.

The change didn't arrive with explanation.

It didn't need to.

It was repeated… adopted… normalized.

And eventually, accepted.

And maybe that's the point.

The snake has long unsettled people. It doesn't move in straight lines. It doesn't announce itself.

It disappears… sheds… returns altered.

It has always represented something unpredictable: something capable of harm... or healing... depending on who's handling it.

Ancient cultures didn't choose it because it was comforting.
They chose it because it was honest.

And once I understood that, I couldn't help but wonder what that quiet transition meant and what it suggested about the symbol's place in the present.

When I designed the cover, I wanted the emblem faded and fractured - to reflect the strained relationship between the identities traced in this book and the medical community.

A visible crack in trust.

What I didn't expect was that the design would surface something deeper: not just tension between people and medicine, but a warning embedded in the symbol itself.

Not just tension between people and medicine... but a warning embedded in the symbol itself.

What made me pause was the presence of the snakes.

After digging a little deeper, I realized my questions weren't about design at all.
They were about inheritance.

Because what this book has shown, again and again, is that the danger was never the tool.

It was the hand using it.

The belief that knowledge grants access. That authority replaces accountability. That progress justifies cost.

We have seen what happens when that belief goes unchecked.

Bodies taken. Voices dismissed. Communities studied, managed, corrected... but rarely protected.

Not in the dark.

Not in the past.

Here.

Now.

And still, we are asked to trust. To sign. To consent. To believe that what stands in front of us now is fundamentally different from what came before.

Sometimes it is.

Sometimes it isn't.

And the difference is not always made clear.

This is what lingers.

Not fear.

Not rejection.

Awareness.

Because forgetting and understanding are not the same thing.

Even when systems do not.

So, the question is no longer whether harm has happened.

We've answered that. Repeatedly.

The question is whether we recognize it when it looks cleaner, when it sounds better, when it comes with credentials... and a signature line at the bottom of the page.

The symbol didn't change by accident.
And neither did the systems built around it.

So don't just look at it.

Understand it.
Question it.

And more importantly...

pay attention to the hands that carry it.

It doesn't always look like history.

Sometimes it looks like a form... the very one we started with.

A few questions you're expected to answer... but cannot.

A line at the bottom...

asking for your signature.

Because history has never needed darkness to repeat itself…

only permission.

Sources & Further Reading

The stories in this book are rooted in lived experience, cultural memory, and the patterns history has tried to soften or erase.

What follows is the evidence beneath that silence - the research, records, reporting, and scholarship that support the truths carried through these pages.

These sources do not replace the narrative; they reveal the ground it stands on.

Night Doctors & Louisiana Skulls

1. **Washington, Harriet A.** *Medical Apartheid: The Dark History of Medical Experimentation on Black Americans from Colonial Times to the Present.* Doubleday, 2007.
2. **Savitt, Todd L.** "The Use of Blacks for Medical Experimentation and Demonstration in the Old South." *The Journal of Southern History*, vol. 48, no. 3, 1982, pp. 331–48.
3. **Washington, Harriet A.** "Medical Apartheid." *American Medical Association Journal of Ethics*, vol. 14, no. 6, 2012, pp. 537–46.
4. **Bunn, Curtis.** "University Returns Remains of Enslaved People Taken from New Orleans' Charity Hospital." *NBC News*, 29 May 2025.

5. **Leipzig University.** "University Returns Human Remains Taken from Enslaved People in New Orleans." *Leipzig University Press Release*, 6 June 2025.

HENRIETTA LACKS & HELA CELLS

1. **Skloot, Rebecca.** *The Immortal Life of Henrietta Lacks*. Crown Publishers, 2010.
2. **"The Legacy of Henrietta Lacks."** *Johns Hopkins Medicine*, johnshopkinsmedicine.org.
3. **Beskow, Laura M.** "Lessons from HeLa Cells: The Ethics and Policy of Governing Human Tissue Samples." *Annual Review of Genomics and Human Genetics*, vol. 17, 2016, pp. 395–416.
4. **Callaway, Ewen.** "HeLa Publication Brews Bioethical Storm." *Nature*, 23 Mar. 2013.
5. **Kemet, Shakkaura.** "Insight Medicine Lacks — The Continuing Relevance of Henrietta Lacks." *The New England Journal of Medicine*, 29 Aug. 2019.

TUSKEGEE SYPHILIS STUDY

1. **Jones, James H.** *Bad Blood: The Tuskegee Syphilis Experiment*. Free Press, 1993.
2. **"The Tuskegee Timeline."** *Centers for Disease Control and Prevention*, cdc.gov.
3. **"Tuskegee Syphilis Study Administrative Records."** *U.S. National Archives*, archives.gov.

4. **Clinton, Bill.** "Remarks in Apology to African Americans on the Tuskegee Study." *The White House*, 16 May 1997.
5. **Brandt, Allan M.** "Racism and Research: The Case of the Tuskegee Syphilis Study." *Hastings Center Report*, vol. 8, no. 6, Dec. 1978, pp. 21–29.

Puerto Rico Pill Trials

1. **Briggs, Laura.** *Reproducing Empire: Race, Sex, Science, and U.S. Imperialism in Puerto Rico*. University of California Press, 2002.
2. **Ramírez de Arellano, Annette B., and Conrad Seipp.** *Colonialism, Catholicism, and Contraception: A History of Birth Control in Puerto Rico*. University of North Carolina Press, 1983.
3. **Tone, Andrea.** *Devices and Desires: A History of Contraceptives in America*. Hill and Wang, 2001.
4. **"The Birth Control Pill: A History."** *PBS American Experience*, pbs.org.
5. **López, Iris.** *Matters of Choice: Puerto Rican Women's Struggle for Reproductive Freedom*. Rutgers University Press, 2008.

Native American Sterilization

1. **Lawrence, Jane.** "The Indian Health Service and the Sterilization of Native American Women." *American Indian Quarterly*, vol. 24, no. 3, Summer 2000, pp. 400–19.

2. **U.S. General Accounting Office.** *Investigation of Allegations Concerning Indian Health Service*. 4 Nov. 1976.
3. **Smith, Andrea.** *Conquest: Sexual Violence and American Indian Genocide*. South End Press, 2005.
4. **Torpy, Sally J.** "Native American Women and Coerced Sterilization: On the Trail of Tears in the 1970s." *American Indian Culture and Research Journal*, vol. 24, no. 2, 2000, pp. 1–22.
5. **"Reproductive Justice and Native Women."** *Native American Rights Fund*, narf.org.

Asian Communities

1. **Lee, Erika.** *The Making of Asian America: A History*. Simon & Schuster, 2015.
2. **Rich, Motoko.** "Japan Apologizes for Forced Sterilizations Under Eugenics Law." *The New York Times*, 24 May 2019.
3. **"Japan Passes Law Compensating Victims of Forced Sterilization."** *BBC News*, 24 Apr. 2019.
4. **"Japanese American Incarceration: Health and Medical Care."** *Densho Encyclopedia*, encyclopedia.densho.org.

Appalachia

1. **Macy, Beth.** *Dopesick: Dealers, Doctors, and the Drug Company That Addicted America*. Little, Brown and Company, 2018.

2. **Stoll, Steven.** *Ramp Hollow: The Ordeal of Appalachia*. Hill and Wang, 2017.
3. **Goodnough, Abby.** "OxyContin Maker Purdue Pharma Pleads Guilty to Federal Drug Charges." *The New York Times*, 21 Oct. 2020.
4. **"Health Disparities in Appalachia."** *Appalachian Regional Commission*, 2017.
5. **Quinones, Sam.** *Dreamland: The True Tale of America's Opiate Epidemic*. Bloomsbury, 2015.

White Bodies, White Data

1. **Criado Perez, Caroline.** *Invisible Women: Data Bias in a World Designed for Men*. Abrams Press, 2019.
2. **Sjoding, Michael W., et al.** "Racial Bias in Pulse Oximetry Measurement." *The New England Journal of Medicine*, 17 Dec. 2020.
3. **Vyas, Darshali A., et al.** "Hidden in Plain Sight — Reconsidering the Use of Race Correction in Clinical Algorithms." *The New England Journal of Medicine*, 27 Aug. 2020.
4. **"Racial and Ethnic Disparities in Maternal Outcomes."** *American College of Obstetricians and Gynecologists*, acog.org.
5. **Nelson, Alondra.** *The Social Life of DNA: Race, Reparations, and Reconciliation After the Genome*. Beacon Press, 2016.

What Carries Forward

1. **"Finding Your Roots."** ***PBS***
2. **Nelson, Alondra.** *The Social Life of DNA: Race, Reparations, and Reconciliation After the Genome.* Beacon Press, 2016.
3. **"African American Genealogy Resources."** *BlackPast*, blackpast.org.

Diagnosis & Discovery

1. **"Sickle Cell Trait."** *Centers for Disease Control and Prevention*, cdc.gov.
2. **Ashley-Koch, Allison, et al.** "Sickle Hemoglobin Allele and Sickle Cell Disease: A HuGE Review." *American Journal of Epidemiology*, vol. 151, no. 9, 2000, pp. 839–45.
3. **Naik, Rakhi P., and Vence L. Bonham.** "Sickle Cell Trait: A Complex and Potentially Underappreciated Carrier State." *JAMA*, 20 Sept. 2016.
4. **"Hydrocephalus Fact Sheet."** *National Institute of Neurological Disorders and Stroke*, ninds.nih.gov.
5. **"Hydrocephalus."** *American Association of Neurological Surgeons*, aans.org.

Modern Echoes – COVID Era

1. **"COVID-19 Racial and Ethnic Health Disparities."** *Centers for Disease Control and Prevention*, cdc.gov.
2. **Hooper, Monica Webb, et al.** "COVID-19 and Racial/Ethnic Disparities." *JAMA*, 23 June 2020.

3. **Eligon, John, et al.** "Black Americans Face Alarming Rates of Coronavirus Infection in Some States." *The New York Times*, 7 Apr. 2020.
4. **Price-Haywood, Eboni G., et al.** "Hospitalization and Mortality Among Black Patients and White Patients with COVID-19." *The New England Journal of Medicine*, 25 June 2020.
5. **Khazanchi, Rohan, et al.** "Racism, Not Race, Drives Inequity Across the COVID-19 Continuum." *JAMA Network Open*, Sept. 2020.

Thank you for reading *Marked by History*

Every book begins with a question.

This one asked what happens when family stories, medical histories, and cultural memory collide.

Other questions led to other stories.

Scan below to explore more books and projects from

Cathy R. Foreman.

www.ingramcontent.com/pod-product-compliance
Lightning Source LLC
LaVergne TN
LVHW090854250926
848801LV00035B/36